D1641479

Adrian Spârlac is the author of *Alzheimer's Return to Functionality* and *Essay on the Classification of Human Traditional Senses*. He has a Bachelor of Science degree in Psychology. What made him to write this piece of work is the highly intriguing fact that memory has a sequential or episodical return to a patient suffering from Alzheimer's disease. That led him to draw the conclusion that in Alzheimer's disease, memory is intact but for certain reasons it is not accessed. The author of this book will reveal some of those reasons among other highly engaging and very interesting things that our readers will come across in this new piece of work.

This book is dedicated to all the people who are helping others driven by their inner force based upon their ethical and moral values.

Adrian Spârlac

ALZHEIMER'S RETURN TO FUNCTIONALITY

AUSTIN MACAULEY PUBLISHERS™

LONDON · CAMBRIDGE · NEW YORK · SHARJAH

Copyright © Adrian Spârlac (2020)

The right of Adrian Spârlac to be identified as author of this work has been asserted by him in accordance with section 77 and 78 of the Copyright, Designs and Patents Act 1988.

All rights reserved. No part of this publication may be reproduced, stored in a retrieval system, or transmitted in any form or by any means, electronic, mechanical, photocopying, recording, or otherwise, without the prior permission of the publishers.

Any person who commits any unauthorised act in relation to this publication may be liable to criminal prosecution and civil claims for damages.

This book is not intended as a substitute for consultation with a licensed healthcare practitioner. Before you begin any healthcare program, or change your lifestyle in anyway, you will consult your physician or another licensed healthcare practitioner to ensure that you are in good health and that the examples contained in this book will not harm you. This book provides content related to physical and/or mental health issues. As such, use of this book implies your acceptance of this disclaimer.

A CIP catalogue record for this title is available from the British Library.

ISBN 9781528979832 (Paperback)
ISBN 9781528979849 (Hardback)
ISBN 9781528979863 (ePub e-book)

www.austinmacauley.com

First Published (2020)
Austin Macauley Publishers Ltd
25 Canada Square
Canary Wharf
London
E14 5LQ

The author wishes to express his gratitude and special thanks to Daniela from Be Social Events Inc., Toronto, Canada and Austin Macauley Publishers from United Kingdom of Great Britain who made the publishing of this book possible.

Table of Contents

"Strengthen your body by labour, and your mind through study."

– Socrates

Introduction

We chose to begin the introduction of this work with the wisdom quote from the philosophy of the great Greek philosopher Socrates by which it tells us very clearly what we have to do in order to keep ourselves in good shape, both physically and mentally, for as long as possible.

This idea was later taken up by the Romans who in their turn said, *"Mens sana in corpore sano."* Which means in Latin 'a healthy mind in a healthy body'. It is not for nothing that the Romans have put the mind before the body which makes us believe that they have perceived the mental power as being above the physical. Today's science can only strengthen the knowledge of the Romans about this phenomenon because on particular occasions, it has been demonstrated that the mind of man plays a very important role in his own healing even from particularly grave diseases, but at the same time, it can kill him as well.

That being said, it does not mean that we have to make a discrepancy between mind and body, but they must always be taken together. Expressing one through the other in optimal parameters reflects the harmony of individual functionality.

We hope that this work will have what it takes to open up new perspectives for assessment and support in the best interest of patients, and the enrichment of the knowledge in this field across the world as well.

During this work, we will present what dementia is in general; we will talk about the typology and the differences between them, and an original approach on the casuistry which is very important indeed. Further in this book, we will also describe through original ideas how memory can be affected by certain forms of dementia.

This work also proposes a theoretical approach from our perspective on the causes and mechanisms that produce this disease, about which is not known enough at the moment to be able actually to heal patients, but slowing down the process of its degeneration only.

This book has two main extremely bold objectives:

1. Demonstration by logical, practical and case studies that memory in Alzheimer's disease is always ready to be functional again being accessed by the mechanisms involved, the phenomenon being episodic with the specification that in time, the distance between the episodes is increasing. Here, memory is not the problem that periodically recurs to the patient but the progressive failure of its access mechanisms and ability to form new memories.

2. There are clear evidences that brain shrinkage does not necessarily cause dementia.
   The reason we are writing this book is because of a very intriguing fact about Alzheimer's disease, mainly, the sequential return of memory in the sufferers from this illness which we should call them mental awakenings. Those awakenings give us the hope to believe that there is a way for the patients of returning to their functionality if we help, somehow, directly or indirectly the mechanisms of memory recollection.

"First, do no harm."

– Hippocrates

"Second, do some good."

– Anne M Lipton

Chapter I. Dementia

1.1 Dementia Throughout European History

Dementia was still mentioned in antiquity by the great thinkers of those times, and the first descriptions on the European continent were made by Hippocrates (460–370 BC), which were merely statements made on the basis of observations on symptomatology. The Father of Medicine considered that mental imbalance even death was due to the imbalance of humours. He had distinguished four humours responsible for the personality of man, such as blood, lymph, yellow gall and black gall. He was also the first who wrote about the presence of cerebrospinal fluid in the brain calling it 'water that surrounds the brain'. We will be talking about this very important thing later in our work.

Plato (427–347 BC on his true name Aristocles because Plato has his nickname due to his broad chest, so in English would sound like Chesty) went further on Hippocrates' ideas, stating that when acid or bitter humour crosses the body and intervenes in the movements of the soul mingling with it, it causes inconveniences that vary in intensity and resemble prostration or oblivion.

On his turn, Aristotle (381–322 BC), being a student of Plato and later Alexander the Great's (356–323 BC) teacher, indicates that memory loss is due exclusively to physical affections, as the ancient Egyptians said that all diseases regardless of manifestation had a physical cause.

Thus, he sets forth two ideas that stand up even today, namely: Mental decline is directly proportional to aging and old age itself is a kind of illness. Because we have mentioned earlier such a great personality as Alexander, we could not resist the temptation to share with our readers another possibility regarding the reason why the greatest commander of all time went with is quest beyond Persia. Most people say that was driven by his personal ambition, but it could be something else based on the fact that he always wanted to see things for himself. As we said earlier, Aristotle was his teacher, and he was taught among many other things that earth was a disc-shaped planet, and after India, it should be the end of the planet. That was the paradigm at the time about the shape of our planet in ancient Greece that lasted in Europe until the renaissance.

Alexander, at the beginning of his campaign against mighty Persia which it was the military super power at that moment, was driven by ambition, indeed, but after that, was driven by curiosity, and was eager to know the truth. He wanted to see for himself the end of the earth which lied beyond India, and verify Aristotle's teachings if were right about the shape of our planet. That was the reason that lied, we believe, behind his quest beyond Persia and perhaps not the ambition of conquering the world as it is widely considered but the thirst for knowledge.

Eventually, Alexander had to stop advancing in his quest at the request of his generals being tired of fighting for so many years, reminding him, at last, of a promise he made to them at the beginning of campaign that he will not lead them as a tyrant but as a friend, so he had to listen to them, and keep his promise despite the fact that he was not far away from knowing the truth that's why he did not want to give up his quest so easily.

Returning to our main subject, after a brief incursion on Alexander the Great's campaign, through the ideas of Aristotle, the medical vision has been influenced by establishing that the decrease in mental capacities is primarily related to aging.

Regarding the above idea indicated by Aristotle which, in fact, was the medical paradigm of the Egyptians at the time stating that all diseases regardless of manifestation had a physical cause obliges us to bring some of the stories less known to large public of another great Greek personality called Socrates (470–399 BC).

While in the army, Socrates got to know a Thracian medic, and he learned about their paradigm of healing from them. He was told that Zamolxes (or Zalmoxis) teachings, which was God and king of Thracians (a sort of Dalai Lama of Tibet), does not try to heal the eyes without healing the head or the head without taking the body in to account in the same way the body cannot be healed without the soul. That was the problem with the Greek doctors, the Thracians said, for not being able to heal many illnesses because they were not considering the part of a whole but only the part itself, and if the whole is not feeling well, then the part will not feel fine either. He emphasised that everything comes from within the soul that's why it is very important to take good care of the soul in order to heal the head or the body. That kind of thinking was actually forming the platform of later Gestalt psychology founded and developed in 1890 by the famous Austrian philosopher Christian von Ehrenfels (1859–1932). Probably being a philosopher and having red Socrates, Plato or Euripides stories regarding the Thracians' ideology on medicine got him the idea of gestalt. Talking about philosophy…in the Netherlands around 1980, the philosophy teachers were proclaiming that the history of philosophy began with the Greeks **(Angela Roothaan** in the article **Plato studied in Egypt)**. The question is how did they overlook the stuff about the Thracians written by those prominent Greek personalities mentioned above? We do not have to forget the fact that many of the Greek gods were taken from the Thracians when their religion was polytheistic (believe in multiple gods) like Ares the God of war, Dionysus God of wine and fertility etc. Later, they would change to monotheism through Zalmoxis while the Greeks were still in polytheism until Christianity. The Getae called by Herodotus or Dacians called by the romans were the most righteous and the bravest among the Thracians, the father of history writes about them as having an innate ability towards philosophy.

That was the paradigm of Zalmoxian School of Medicine which, fortunately, more and more is adopted by some of the greatest scientists today. Some of them they heard about it, others got at this level of thinking by themselves. Thracians even had an oath much earlier than Hippocrates that had to be sworn at the graduation which it can be reconstituted from Plato's writings.

Hippocrates himself knew about that Thracian oath because one of his medicine teachers was a famous Thracian doctor called Herodicus of Selymbria whose theories are considered to be the fundaments of sports medicine. Even back then, Herodicus knew the importance of walking for the health benefit and recommended to his patients to do so everyday a distance of 20 miles...such things we only heard recently how healthy walking is. So Hippocrates took the Thracian oath of medicine which was a **moral commitment** to the profession of medics and updated it as we know it today. We have to mention that Thracians peoples were located where now Romania and Bulgaria is today, but their territory was much larger than that. Herodotus (484–425 BC), the father of history and a contemporary of Socrates, made very interesting descriptions of who Thracian people really were, but although very interesting, we will not go now further deeper in ancient history.

On the basis of Zalmoxian School of Medicine and using strong arguments supporting it, we will further show in this work how Alzheimer's is an illness of the whole body, but we will get to that soon.

We continue our incursion into the annals of medical history concerning dementia with Aulus Cornelius Celsus (25 BC to 50 AD) considered to be the Hippocrates of the Romans who was probably the first to use the name dementia, says in his book 'De Medicina' that insanity begins with continuous dementia when the patient, while retaining his senses, nourishes all sorts of imaginations and once installed, the mind will obey them **(NC Berchtold, CW Cotman 1998)**.

The meaning that Celsus attributes to the term 'dementia', in fact, consists of two words, namely de and mentia, where the second means the mind and the first comes from the dispossession, and, therefore, we have the dispossessions of the mind (memory loss) (Latin).

Aretaeus a Cappadocian physician during Roman Emperor Nero speaks of a decrease in the condition of the body as a result of aging that weakens the senses and ultimately affects the mental faculties.

Claudius Galenus (129–216 AD) whom Roman Emperor Marcus Aurelius called '*Primum sane medicorum esse philosophorum autem solum*' meaning the first among the doctors and unique among philosophers, looked at old age as a step between health and illness and that memory loss indicated senility. With old age begins alteration of the brain and can no longer keep perceptions on the long-term.

A very interesting principle, which continues to exist today, was even put forward by Marcus Tullius Cicero (106–43 BC), namely that a responsible, active life full of intellectual challenges can prevent degeneration. He did not regard old age as a disease but as a course of nature. In his understanding, senility touches only people with weak characters and trivial preoccupations.

Cicero recommends a constant training of memory which is essential in the prevention of early dementia. It can successfully fight against aging by focussing on cognitive exercises, through permanent challenges to thought and understanding. Yet despite these beneficial tips, one cannot avoid the encounter with death.

Once with the inevitable passage of time in the Middle Ages, things have taken an ugly turn in what concerns dementia sufferers. Let us not forget the fact that at that time, Christianity was the governing force of the whole European continent, and that ideology over people with mental disorders dominated the power of thinking of most people. Thus, at the time was circulated the idea that the mental sufferers were possessed by the devil; therefore, they were subjected to exorcism 'sessions' enriched with tortures to make the unclean (the devil) go out of their body.

If at the end of these 'sessions' there was no 'healing' of the sufferer, it was proceeding to the 'purification' of the soul, mainly, to burning them alive on the fire stack.

Well, not all of Europe used the above healing methods, each country between the X–XV centuries had its own 'solutions'. So in Germany, they tried to isolate the cases of mental illnesses and locked them in the so-called 'Towers of the Fools', a kind of a hospice which, in fact, weren't nothing else but some gloomy dungeons. In England, they crushed their heads with a hammer *maleus maleficarum* (the hammer of the evildoers, destined for the witches) who would not have had the good fortune to have been taken to Bedlam (Bethlehem Royal Hospital), the oldest European hospital for mentally ill, founded in the year 1377 and operated until 1948. In Byzantium, however, the problem was different, where the sufferers of mental disorders were gathered in *xenodoc*, a combination of the asylum and hospital where they were taking care for by specialised personnel **(Magazin istoric, Apr 1969)**.

The Byzantine approach is due to the interaction between Constantinople and other cultures with more advanced thoughts in medicine such as the Greeks or the Arabs.

With the Arab influence in Europe, the renaissance took place between the fourteenth and seventeenth centuries creating an intellectual explosion of Western Europe that, eventually, among other things led to a better knowledge and understanding of mental affections.

The emergence of psychiatry, a term introduced by German physician Johann Christian Reill (1759–1813) in 1808, opened new perspectives for patient research, diagnosis and support.

Thus, at the beginning of the nineteenth century, with a new branch of medicine dealing with the study and treatment of the psychiatric illnesses that Reill (Goethe's doctor) originally called *Psychiaterie*, it laid the foundations of a modern medical-philosophical approach of mental disorders.

Thus, the French doctor Benedict Morel (1809–1873) in his book *Traite de maladie mentale* (Treaty of Mental Illness) uses for the first time in 1860 the term of *demence precoce* (early dementia in French), later adopted in 1891 by Emil Kraeplin, denoting in Latin *dementia precox* (the precox dementia in Latin) representing the diagnosis of schizophrenia.

Finally, Aloysius Alzheimer (1864–1915) identifies and publishes for the first time the first case of presenile dementia that his colleague Kraeplin called Alzheimer's disease.

1.2 A Brief Look at the Typology of Dementia

Dementia is an irreversible clinical syndrome characterised by the progressive loss or decline of cognitive and mental functions compared to an earlier level.

Dementia generally represents a collection of over fifty forms of brain disease, and the most common types are Alzheimer's, vascular, Lewy body, frontotemporal (Pick's disease), Korsakov and Creutzfeldt-Jakob.

According to the Dutch statistics, one of five people acquire over time one of various forms of dementia, some earlier, around the age of 40 such as frontotemporal dementia, others later around 70 years of age such as Alzheimer's.

So from an epidemiological point of view, statistics generally show us that 5% of the population over 65 have Alzheimer's and the risk increases. With 80 years of age, one in three people is affected by this form of dementia, which is actually the most common, 50% of all cases of dementia **(F Tudose, 2009)**.

Dementia forms differ from each other through casuistic and symptomatology specific to each condition, with the indication that causes are not always known.

We will briefly present in the following few dementia types.

Vascular dementia

It is the most common form of dementia after the Alzheimer's type. The causes of this disease are due to chronic reduction of blood flow to the brain as a result of external physical trauma such as cranial concussions or internal conditions leading to cerebral vascular accidents, but also to the degree of blood viscosity which can, in turn, prevent an optimal circulation of blood to different parts of the brain.

Another cause that we deduced from our research is determined by very low blood pressure in combination with an obstruction of the respiratory system during sleep-provoking apnoea. For a better understanding, apnoea is a sleep disorder characterised by pauses in breathing during sleep.

This prevents the brain from feeding properly with oxygen. The cerebral parts with the highest oxygen consumption due to abundant vascularisation are temporal lobes, and here the effect will be the most pronounced, and as a consequence, will occur in time a decrease and a dysfunction of the brain in these areas which will inevitably lead to the appearance of the first signs of dementia. Here, we have to mention a very important fact that the brain alone uses 20% of the body's oxygen resources.

The degree of impairment is expressed by memory loss in the affected sector, confusion and other signs of dementia.

Lewy body dementia

This form of dementia should be addressed with particular attention when the diagnosis is to be made. This is very difficult due to the symptomatic similarity with Parkinson's disease but also with Alzheimer's when the disease progresses.

Again, we can talk about Lewy body syndrome if specific symptoms occur before or until one year after the diagnosis of Parkinson's disease and analogous when these symptoms of Lewy body dementia occur later on we speak of Parkinson's disease. This is due to the presence of Lewy bodies in both Parkinson's and Alzheimer's. Lewy bodies are formed by an abnormal protein concentration that affects the smooth functioning of neurons in the cerebral cortex and limbic system, the highest concentration being in the *substantia nigra* (black substance in Latin) that is part of the basal ganglia. Without the substantia nigra is not possible to perform movements, so once affected the nerves in this area will cause motor disorders. At the neuronal level, the Lewy corpuscles makes it harder and even blocks the flow of the neurotransmitter called dopamine. Or if communication of a neuron with another is blocked, then this neuron will die. The death of a neuron is called *apoptosis*. At the same time, a disturbance of the dopamine flow between neurons explains the tremor to Parkinson's and Lewy body dementia.

After 45 years of age, the number of neurons from substantia nigra begins to decline significantly at a rate of 1% per year. This is not a problem among healthy people only when the number of neurons has decreased by 20–30% and the process of generating new neurons called neurogenesis has been completely overwhelmed. It is only then that the first symptoms of Parkinson or Lewy body occur, especially because besides this problem is the deficiency of dopamine existing in the rest of the neurons...so double trouble.

Unlike Parkinson's disease, Lewy body dementia may present symptoms as hallucination in which the patient sees objects, animals or even people who are not in his physical presence but with whom he communicates, thus revealing serious behavioural disturbances. Other symptoms that may appear in Lewy body dementia are disorders of alert and attention systems such as gaze into the void for a long time. As in Alzheimer's dementia case, appear cognitive, attention problems, confusion states and ultimately so-called memory loss.

The causes of Lewy body dementia are not known, it is only presumed to be, just as we have intuited that it is related to Alzheimer's or Parkinson's due to the presence of Lewy corpuscles in all forms of dementia.

Frontotemporal dementia (Pick's disease)

Frontotemporal dementia is also called Pick's disease due to the fact that in 1892, German psychiatrist Arnold Pick describes for the first time such form of dementia of a 71-year-old patient. He noticed that both the prefrontal cortex and the temporal lobes seemed diminished in size, and in these areas, were recorded portions of dead cells. In the same brain parts, the remaining portions were full of swellings, these were called Pick cells. However, in most cases of frontotemporal dementia, these Pick cells are missing; therefore, the name of this type of illness is unanimously accepted as frontotemporal dementia.

This form of dementia occurs more often among patients aged about 40 years. Behavioural disorders are the first signs of this disease, the affected areas are the prefrontal cortex and temporal lobes, areas responsible with emotions, cognition, behaviour, decision and language.

Symptomatically, Pick's disease is divided into three stages:

- Changes in behaviour, personality and emotional disturbances.
- Language disorders, echolalia (repetition of another person's spoken words) and progressive aphasia (impairment of language), at some point, the patient will no longer be able to speak anymore but will still be able to understand what he is told.
- Motor disorders, problems with walking, maintaining balance, coordination of movements and trembling.

One important thing to mention in this form of dementia is that memory disturbances occur later in most cases.

It is believed that the causality of this form of dementia is thought to be the Tau protein that can no longer ensure the axonal stability of the neuron, thereby affecting its proper functioning.

This dysfunction of the protein may be due to a genetic mutation or a set of external factors exerted over a prolonged period of time depending on the limits of each organism such as:

- Lack of vitamins
- Extreme stress over a long period of time or chronic stress
- Social isolation
- Lack of motion
- Lack of affection

We will show during this work the functioning of this protein on neuronal axonal structures.

It is worth mentioning that in over 40% of cases, the frontotemporal dementia is inherited. The chances of acquiring this disease are ½ if one of the parents has this illness. If the heir does not become ill, due to the inherited chromosomal 'strength' from the healthy parent it will become a carrier of the dysfunctional protein.

The chromosome is a cell with the role of properly preserving and transmitting hereditary information to the daughter cell by the process called mitosis. Through mitosis, the continuity of a species, the growth and development of the individual, as well as the repair of the tissues in case of diseases, are ensured **(C Stanciu, 2014)**.

It should be noted that the self-repairing capabilities of the organism is unfortunately limited; otherwise, it would mean not only to be immortal, but we will not know either the disease or the old age. Well, here is something interesting we want to bring to our readers attention regarding the longevity of mankind described in the Bible. In the beginning, people used to live much longer like Adam, for instance, he used to live 930 years, Seth lived 913 years, Enosh 905, Kenan 910, Methuselah 969, Noah 950 years etc. After that, Noah people's longevity decreased, so his son Shem lived 600 years, Arpachshad 438, Shelah 433, Peleg 464 etc. Later on, Abraham lived 175 years, Sarah his wife 127 years, Ishmael 137, Isaac 180 etc. so we see a new decreasing in ages.

The last decrease in ages decided by God was to be around 120 years old, and all that for demographical reasons. *"And the Lord said: My spirit will not be in man forever, for he is only flesh, so the days of his life will be a hundred and twenty years."* In a prayer of Moses it is written that: *"Our days may come to seventy years or eighty, if our strength endures."* So this is the most common age people were reaching in Moses' time and pretty much the same remained in our days.

Now comes the question, would not the decreasing in age, which it did not happen in one go, have something to do with the decrease of the self-repairing capabilities of the cells at the DNA level? Wouldn't be God influencing, somehow, those particular cells? It is a possibility.

In conclusion, the explanation of this phenomenon such as living for several centuries is according to what has been said above in relation to the extremely efficient individual chromosomal self-repair capacity for such a long time. Of course, there is another self-repair system present in our organism, and that is the endocrine system, but the most important role played in extreme longevity of humans like the Bible figures mentioned on the other page of our work is determined by chromosomal self-repair capacity at the DNA level. Okay, but such powerful chromosomal repair system has to be matched by a formidable energy supply at the cell level. That brings our thoughts towards ***mitochondrion*** which can be considered the powerhouse of a cell. What if God made a succession of changes at the level of cell energy like giving less power in the 'batteries'? And why mitochondrial DNA in humans is transmitted from one parent only, which is the woman? This is one of the reasons considered by scientists that explains why women live longer than men **(BBC article – Fruit flies offer DNA clue to why women live longer, 2012)**. To make the equation simple, the amount of energy produced by a cell influences the efficiency of repair system at cell level over time. Just like an old tape recorder on batteries, for example, in the beginning, the sound was correct until the low-level energy in the battery was reached, after that, we could hear the distortions of the sound that become worse and worse until it stops…a living organism works pretty much on the same principle. Aging is a sign that low battery energy has been reached and all begins from the interior of the body at the cell level, and well, at a certain point, we are beginning to notice that. So metaphorically speaking, perhaps God changed our old long-life batteries (expensive) with newer not so long-life batteries (cheaper) for demographical reasons.

However, we are not absolutely certain that extreme longevity was applied to whole mankind or only to Adam and Eve descendants exclusively, although there are many legends in many different countries around the globe about people living extremely long. We are certainly aware that what we are about to say will contravene with the idea of most religious believers. Adam and Eve were not the first humans made by God because He already made humans before them as we can understand from the readings of the Bible. Humans were created both masculine and feminine. And they already lived in communities and lands before Adam and Eve. Okay, here we have to make sure things are not misinterpreted of what we are saying, it is not written with the following words in the Bible: *"God made people before Adam and Eve,"* but trough deduction, we cannot suppose, otherwise, that indeed were people around before Adam and Eve. The strongest argument of this idea is given by the story of the elder son of Adam and Eve, Cain.

After Cain killed his brother Abel, had to leave the place as God ordered him to do, so, therefore, he got scared that anyone who would find him would kill him. Well…by whom was he afraid of since there were no other people around as most religious people believe? Further, it is clearly written in the Bible that Cain went to a land at east of Eden called Nod, and there he had his own family. Well…how could he have a family if there were no other people on earth as most Christians believe; besides, he left alone the place where he used to live with his parents Adam and Eve. On the other hand, there are human skeletons found on different parts of the world dated back millions years ago in Australia, Ethiopia and so on. However, the Jewish calendar Seder Olam Rabbah, which is the oldest calendar that is still in use today, began with the creation of Adam and Eve which is placed in 3761 BC and Noah's flood in 2015 BC but other sources indicate the year of creation being at 3950 BC, other 3982 BC or 4004 BC and the flood at 2348 BC according to James Ussher' chronology and as you see there is no big difference. All these being said, we figure that Adam and Eve were made around 5781 years ago, and the oldest human skeleton found is millions of years old, so the conclusion is clear, there were people around before Adam. Considering the above arguments, we conclude that it is not certain if such a long longevity was granted for the whole mankind or for Adam and Eve's descendants only, but as we have pointed out on the previous page, there are, indeed, legends about people living for so long in other cultures as well like: in Sumer, King Gilgamesh had ruled 126 years and met Utnapishtim which it could be Noah if we look at the similarity of story and the time when Noah lived in, it is possible that Noah and Gilgamesh met according to Sumerian poems.

Sumerian calendar had 354 days divided in 12 months, and once in a couple of years, they were adding another month to make up for the remaining 11 days…so is not a big difference with our calendar today. In India, Persia, China, Japan, Greece and many more, they all had advanced cultures whose calendar was almost or just as accurate as our calendar today, so what if it is true for these people to live that long? If they would have a much more efficient chromosomal repair system supported by a magnificent energy cell supply from a much better mitochondria, it would, indeed, be possible to live that long, but we will leave this very interesting subject to our readers reasoning to decide, and we will return to our main topic of this work concluding with the words full of wisdom of General Mircea Chelaru: *"Science…is God's urge for people to come closer to Him."*

Coming back to our previous idea, each body has its own individual cellular repair capabilities, but some things cannot be repaired by its own chromosomal system, and the body becomes the carrier of certain abnormalities that will be passed on to the offspring, and, eventually, they can benefit from a genetic repair from the part of the healthy parent as we said earlier.

Even if that inherited and the individual is 'solved', he will not experience symptoms of dementia, but it will still have a weakness in his own DNA link, which, in turn, will transmit it further.

When one of his heirs in the next generations will have a partner with a weakness of the same nature, the onset of dementia or another type of illness will be inevitable in their newborn, only that the symptoms will appear later.

At the same time, these people may develop a form of dementia due to their sensitivity to the external factors enumerated in one of the previous pages. In other words, the genetic vulnerability being already present, the body expects only the triggering factor from the external environment to be highlighted.

In other order of ideas, we have described some types of dementia so far, but after causality, we categorise them as follows:

- Vascular dementia
- Geriatric dementia (as a result of natural aging)
- Toxic dementia (due to excessive levels of drugs, alcohol, drugs etc.)
- Infectious dementia (syphilis, AIDS etc.)
- Dementias due to internal conditions (tumours, hormonal disturbances vitamin deficiencies, cellular deficiencies etc.), here comes Alzheimer's, Frontotemporal and Lewy body
- Traumatic dementias (blows to the head or isolation of the subject on the long-term)
- Digital dementia (due to excessive use of the computer, will have repercussions on the memory) **(M Spitzer, 2013)**

We believe it is very important to note that ***dementia does not cause brain shrinking, but that brain shrinkage can lead to dementia, and this only under certain circumstances. And the location where the first atrophy of the brain will occur, early symptoms may be revealed.***

These symptoms are different from each other due to the fact that different parts of the brain are affected provided that each part of the brain has its own function which may be manifested trough behaviour. Hence, we conclude that dementia is the disease with over 50 faces.

The principle of brain atrophy after which extends to other parts of the brain is simple, mainly, *each part of the brain communicates with another; once a part of the brain will be affected by atrophy, it will implicitly affect the other parts as well because they will, in turn, no longer be used at the initial parameters.* In other words, a true principle of domino. The physiological mode of functioning of the brain is similar to that of the muscles: if a muscle is not being used, it will get atrophied. Analogously, the brain or its parts, if not used due to certain conditions, will suffer atrophy at some extent. On the other hand, shrinkage of the brain is a symptom of old age, but that does not mean necessarily that memory will become impaired. There are cases of individuals over 80 years old having similar brain shrinkage as an Alzheimer patient and has no memory problems at all.

"Memory is the mother of wisdom."

– Aeschylus

Chapter II. Alzheimer's Dementia

2.1 Characteristics and Aetiology of Alzheimer's Disease

As we have established in the previous chapter, Alzheimer's is part of the dementia group caused by internal conditions as a result of a set of external deficiencies such as lack of vitamins, movement, contact and social affection etc. Once this disease is acquired, it will be taken up in the genetic sequences of the body, and will become hereditary.

This disease is also part of the hereditary group, facts that happens according to the genetic principle described in the previous chapter.

Alzheimer's disease begins long before the first symptoms of dementia occurs, it is about 20 years before the first symptoms appear, and after that, worsens rapidly and progressively culminating with death of the patient after about 10 years of suffering. When the first symptoms appear, the brain structures are already largely affected, and any medication cannot have the desired efficacy and efficiency.

During this period of about 30 years, genetic changes are required to make this anomaly hereditary.

Suppose an individual has Alzheimer's disease, and he will have a baby. If this child also has Alzheimer's, the manifestations of this dementia will not occur earlier than the biological decline of the body, so up to 45 years. So far, no symptomatic Alzheimer's case has been reported in a younger person than 45-year-old.

The latest techniques, although still in the experimental phase, are very promising in blood analysis through which the existence and even the predisposition of the individual for Alzheimer's disease can be detected very early.

We will present below the experiment made by American scientists at the Banner Alzheimer's Institute in Arizona under the guidance of Dr Eric M Reiman to study genetic baggage in relation to Alzheimer's disease.

For this, a group of 44 young people between the ages of 18 and 26 was invited to the experiment. They have carried out various blood tests, cerebrospinal fluid and an MRI scan of the brain.

The results showed that in 20 of them, a mutagenic gene called Presenilin-1 (PSEN1) was found. Under these circumstances, triggering Alzheimer's disease in them is a fact at a certain point.

There was no evidence of the presence of this gene in the other 24 subjects. It should be noted that none of the 44 subjects had symptoms of dementia or cognitive impairment during research.

Researchers, however, noticed differences in the brain structure and functionality of those carrying the mutagenic gene comparative to the non-carriers. Thus, the mutagenic gene carriers had a much higher activity recorded in the hippocampus area than the others. Another difference is a lower amount of grey matter in PSEN1 group than in the others.

In addition, a higher amount of Beta-Amyloid was recorded in the PSEN1 gene carrier group indicating higher amyloid production. The problem exacerbates when this super-production of beta-amyloid begins to deposit and form plaques, and this way, blocking neuronal communication. These plaques were first observed by Aloysius Alzheimer himself.

At present, these beta-amyloid plaque formations is considered to be the basis of Alzheimer's causal disease.

On average, the first symptoms of Alzheimer's disease in PSEN1 gene carriers occurred around the age of 45, demonstrating that the biological marker can be detected 20 years before, appropriate age for a possible treatment.

In conclusion, Dr Eric Reiman says the following: these observations suggest that long before the clinical onset of Alzheimer's disease was already recorded, brain structures are already altered, right before the formation of beta-amyloid plaques. This raises new questions about the change in brain structure and the approach to preventive therapies. Further research on this is needed **(Daily mail telegraph 6/11/2012)**.

In Alzheimer's disease, we observe within the affected neurons, the so-called neurofibrillary tangles (in an entangled shape) of Tau hyperphosphorylated protein. Also, between the neurons, we see beta-amyloid plaques. It is worth mentioning that this highly soluble Tau protein is actually a phosphoprotein, phosphorylation being nothing but the process of adding phosphorus to the neuron. In other words, the Tau phosphoprotein can become phosphorus overcharged through its own phosphorylation process and, therefore, may get overstressed and become entangled. When phosphorus overcharging occurs, that does not mean necessarily that is too much phosphorus in the body but a malfunction at cell level.

Tau protein plays a very important role in stability of the microtubules of the neuron's axon. Microtubules are involved in maintaining the structure of a cell and plays an important role in mitosis and meiosis (asexual and sexual chromosome separation respectively) as well.

In this case, the structure of the axon is not properly maintained because the Tau protein is not ensuring the stability of the microtubules because it has become instable for being entangled due to hyperphosphorylation.

Phosphorus is an essential mineral primarily used for growth and repair of body cells and tissues. Also plays a very important role in energy productions.

The neuronal membrane has a higher content of phospholipids (60%) than the membranes of other cells, and their fluidity is more sensitive to the action of influence factors such as liposoluble substances, temperature etc. **(C Stanciu 2009)**.

The causality and processes of formation of Tau protein entangling within the neuron are not yet known, so we presume and assume that another cause could be a glucose deficiency in rapport with intraneuronal stress as well.

Glucose is the main source of energy for cells that are part of the central nervous system; 25% of glucose is consumed by the brain only, so any anomaly at this level has an effect on the psyche which makes it visible in the individual's behaviour more precisely on self-control and decision-making.

Glucose alone cannot enter neuronal cells except through insulin produced by the pancreas. This is where the following question may arise: can Alzheimer's disease be related to the pancreas?

The answer is yes, but we cannot say with certainty that the pancreas is the main cause...but is just one of the many possibilities because just as well it could be from the liver where the glucose is being produced and stored, and if something goes wrong there...Alzheimer's disease has numerous causes that's why it is so difficult to treat...in our opinion is like curing cancer, but it is to be cured...maybe not yet, but it certainly will. Here, we have to mention that it would depend on the extent of the brain damage in relation to age because the repair capabilities of the brain may not be able to cope with.

For a better understanding of what we will support in the lines to be written in this work, we will give the following example similar to what is happening at the neuron level:

A copper wire that is used for electricity conduction has an insulating protective coating made of plastic or rubber. This insulating coating has a certain thickness depending on the maximum electrical charge the copper wire can carry. If the electrical charge exceeds the parameters at which the wire was calculated, it will become hot, will become red, and the insulating coating will, eventually, melt away from the conducting wire.

With this simplified example, we return to what we said earlier applying this principle to neuronal dimensions.

Stress (the electrical charge) if it exceeds the maximum strength of the neuron will trigger a chain reaction of the following mechanisms:

Glucose, the energy supplier of the neuron, will not be able to cope with the amount of stress caused by hyper nervous excitations, so the phenomenon of so-called *excitotoxicity* occurs.

Then Tau protein, which is present only in the axon and not in the neuron dendrites, will no longer be able to provide the stability and suppleness of the axon tubules which, in this case, is possible that neuronal temperature maybe increased. Prolonged phosphorylation of this protein is maintained thereby exhausting it so badly that it will no longer be able to provide the integrity of the protective layer of the axon.

This hyperphosphorylated Tau protein will disintegrate in tangle heads due to the hyper excitability of the neuron, and will come out of the axon because this will be allowed by the elevated temperature at the axonal level which will cause the neuron membrane in this area to dissolve.

We strongly believe that instability caused by high temperature corroborated with detaching and migrating of entangled Tau protein triggers inevitably an excessive flow of beta-amyloid in the brain which, in this case, acts as part of the autoimmune system to combat an infection at this level because it is seen as an infection. This is the mechanism at cell level that explains what leads to Alzheimer's disease in this case.

Phosphorylation on and off of a protein only form the opening and closing mechanism of the information traffic (communications) at the axonal level, so a reversible process.

…The existence of these free communications between the interior and the exterior within the cell would lead to an installation of a thermodynamic equilibrium for the small components, which would seriously impede the existence (of metabolism) and the functioning (excitability) of the neuron. It imposes this way the need for existence of some ways of closing (inactivation) and opening (activation) of their own depending on certain circumstances **(C Stanciu, 2009)**.

From this, we deduce that due to excitotoxicity, cellular energy decreases what makes a Tau protein hyperphosphorylation occur in the neuron's axon.

Of course, millions of neurons are involved in the thinking process so that under extreme stress conditions for a long period of time, many of them will be affected according to the principles above, so the presence of the hyperphosphorylated formations of Tau proteins on the brain becomes visible.

Once with the onset of so-called neuronal disintegration, in this case, the brain compression process begins as a result of so-called neuronal micro damage. Here, we have to mention that shrinking of the brain has many causes as well.

Researchers have determined that the pathology of the Tau protein originates in the hippocampus more precisely in the entorhinal cortex where it extends further to all the brain regions. They are based on one of the features of Alzheimer's disease, mainly, the reduction of the hippocampus in size, which is visible in an MRI scan and in the sectional examination of the brain.

Geriatric (old age) dementia is also generated in the hippocampus but in the gyrus dentatus area where the most neurogenesis occurs. Thus, this area being affected, there will be an imbalance in the relationship between neurogenesis and apoptosis in an overwhelming favour of the last, unfortunately for us.

Once explained, the presence of neurofibrillary tangles in the brain, we are engaging to describe the presence of beta-amyloid protein plaques as well.

The functionality of this beta-amyloid protein is not well known; however, studies on some animals show that its lack in the brain does not lead to any loss of physiological function **(Y Luo, B Bolon, MA Damore, D Fitzpatrick, 2003)**. However, it has been discovered that this protein plays a role in the activation of kinase enzymes **(M Tabaton, X Zhu, G Perry, 2010)**.

These types of enzymes have the role of transferring phosphates from energy-donating cells to a specific substrate of the consuming cell. This process is called **phosphorylation**.

From here, we deduce the following hypothesis…a poor functioning of kinase enzymes deprives the neuron of the necessary energy. Tau protein inside the axon due to lack of required energy will, eventually, on the long-term disintegrate. The hippocampus responds to this energy deficiency due to the malfunctioning of kinase by super-producing beta-amyloid (it is engaged in activating kinase as well) from its entorhinal cortex. Two characteristics of beta-amyloid protein are: sticky and very toxic, precisely because of its presence in very high quantities. It is very important to know that beta-amyloid becomes harmful only in large quantities!

Due to the causes enumerated above BA (Beta-Amyloid) protein reaches the cerebrospinal fluid but also in the interstitial fluid in high quantities.

The cerebrospinal fluid is secreted by the choroid plexus just outside the hippocampus and the production is around 500ml per day. This fluid is refreshed entirely 3–4 times a day in a continuous process, for removal of residuals eliminated from brain cells.

For a better understanding the cerebrospinal fluid acts like a shock absorber when external injuries at the skull level occur. Also it ensures an imponderability state or suspension of the brain equivalent to a mass of around 50 grams giving the fact that total weight of the brain is somewhere around 1500g. Inexistence of this liquid in humans will make the brain impaired by its own weight in this case.

Well, taking into account the quantity and viscous property of the BA protein may exceed the capabilities of refreshing the cerebrospinal fluid properly which will no longer be able to cope efficiently, will facilitate the depositions of the BA protein in plaques. The vigour of the human body being in decline can no longer cope with the bio physiological processes as at 20 years, the energy decreases considerably, that explains why the first symptoms of Alzheimer's occur not earlier than 45 years. Here, cholesterol plays an important role as well in making blood transport more difficult by obstructing the optimum sanguine circulation at capillary level in the central nervous system.

By what we have written so far, the following question arises... *what if recycling of cerebrospinal fluid or interstitial fluid is not done correctly?* In this case, then the concentration of BA that doesn't need to be large can no longer be properly cleared by eliminating organs (liver and kidney) which inevitably initiate its deposition into plaques. This way the increasing concentration of BA becomes harmful to the neuron by corroding its plasmatic membrane.

As we can see, the causes of Alzheimer's are not only diverse, but it can be a mixture of causes in the same time in most cases that leads to this illness. The aetiology of Alzheimer's disease being very diverse, makes it harder for the healing process, which means that different medical, psychological, nutritional, multidisciplinary treatments all together will have to be discovered depending on the causes and very important, will have to be personalised. That means every patient with his own personalised treatment in order to be effectively helped.

This large amount of BA protein severely affects the synapses of neurons that no longer properly exchange information. Synapses are the spaces between neurons where informational exchange between them occurs or to make it easier for our readers, the place where neurons are joining together. A very important breakthrough on this protein was made in 2009 when it was shown that BA production is linked with the circadian rhythm, increasing during the day and decreasing during the night **(JE Kang, MM Lim, JR Bateman, 2009)**. The same research, even the most recent ones, shows that excessive sleeping deprivation of the body leads to the elevation of BA protein production that can hypothetically trigger Alzheimer's disease over time.

So far, we can see that two major problems originate in the entorhinal cortex of the hippocampus, both tauopathy and

BA secretion, with the mention that death of neurons occurs first here. In conclusion, excessive BA secretion in that area could be a consequence of tauopathy as well.

Also, extremely important to know is that in the hippocampus, neurogenesis is taking place as well, in the area called *gyrus dentatus*.

Neurogenesis, this unique feature of the hippocampus is very easily influenced by stress more precisely by the hormone of this factor called *cortisol*. Any reaction to stress makes this hormone present in large amounts in the blood composition and, hence, in the hippocampus as well. The presence of cortisol from the adrenal glands in large quantities for a long period of time in the hippocampus is very damaging to neurogenesis making it difficult or even preventing the formation of new neuronal cells **(R Kahn, 2006)**. One of the worst effects of stress on the brain is that it can increase the risk of Alzheimer's and other forms of dementia. A very important fact we wish to bring here, the hippocampus regulates memory and emotions and plays a role in various emotional disorders. During long periods of stress, the hippocampus decreases in size and that's one of the reasons why people forget a lot, lose their attention and concentration in those circumstances. On the other hand, studies in older mice have shown that by increasing neurogenesis in the hippocampus, memory can be improved according to Australian scientists from the University of Queensland.

However, the problems do not stop there because other structures of the central nervous immune system are triggered. The cells that make up this part of immune system are called *microglia*, the smartest and most fascinating cells in the human body are activated by beta amyloid **(E Solito, M Sastre, 2012)**. Microglia attacks the BA protein plaques, but destroys healthy tissues in the isolation process of the bad cell as well. Here, it would not be a problem, but these plaques are too many and spread throughout the body, and the focal point is in the hippocampus where the highest concentration of microglia is found so a lot of healthy tissue cells will be destroyed and that helps to even greater damage to the brain as a whole.

To make it easier for the reader is like a dentist when is drilling a hole in a tooth treating a caries, a layer of a healthy tissue of the tooth is being removed along with the decayed surface which makes the hole even bigger…just like what microglia does in the brain.

Let's not forget that the microglia is the one that extracts the neuron in case of apoptosis, and the hippocampus is the area where most neurons die, as the case with Alzheimer's disease.

There is so much to say about microglia, its morphic properties, how they communicate with other cells, repair functions, cells and synapses maintenance, how it helps to establish the neural network in the prenatal period as early as the ninth day, an extraordinarily interesting topic which we hope to approach in a future work.

Other roles of the beta-amyloid protein are protection against oxidative stress **(K Zou, JS Gong, K Yanagisawa, 2002)**, regulating the transport of cholesterol **(ZX Yao, V Papadopoulos, 2002)**, functioning as a transcription factor for genetic information in DNA **(B Maloney, DK Lahiri, 2011)**, activation of the above-described kinase enzymes as well as anti-microbial activities, thus a potential immune system factor associated with pre-inflammatory mechanisms **(SJ Soscia, JE Kirby, KJ Washicosky, 2010)**.

Here's how BA protein is involved in genetic operations, and if it causes at this level any genetic transcription error, it will be transmitted on the hereditary line (see explanations on the Presenilin mutagenic gene).

At the same time, the BA protein also acts as part of the immune system, which makes us accept the possibility that its presence in large amounts explains the role of defences against the hyperphosphorylated protein Tau as we said previously. Both entangled Tau protein and BA plaques are always present in Alzheimer's patients, which was first observed by Alois Alzheimer in 1906. Further, as previously shown, in large amounts, BA protein becomes toxic to neurons, which engages another immune cell formation called the microglia that does not attack the BA protein but the plaques formed by it.

Microglia itself cannot stand alone with this torrent of BA plaques, and then another fascinating cells called macrophage (a type of white cell) cells will get involved as well that have the property through their metabolism to become either a 'military' or a repair cell. What happens in the brain of an Alzheimer's patient is like a real civil war between distinct formations of immune system and bad cells, the battlefield being the brain itself, and that as in any armed conflict there are also collateral victims, which, in this case, are represented by the healthy cell tissues in very close proximity of the plaques or other bad cells.

From all written above, we find that several factors lead to BA protein surplus and each of these should be carefully analysed in order to determine the cause and, implicitly, to apply the most effective treatment. From this, we conclude that although BA plaques cause significant brain damage, we must focus on the main cause of the presence in large quantities of BA protein in the brain. This is the key to success (finding the causes) in preventing or treating Alzheimer's or any other disease; otherwise, we will only treat certain symptoms as usually happens in most cases, unfortunately.

In normal aging, BA plaques are in a small number. They are considered pathological in relation to age if their number exceeds:

- Under 50 years – 2 plates / mm^2
- Between 51 and 64 years – 8 plates / mm^2
- Between 65 and 74 years old – 10 plates / mm^2
- Above 75 years – 15 plates / mm^2 **(ZS Khachaturian, 1985, M Covic, T Covic, C Datu, 2007)**.

There is, currently, no medicine to prevent or treat properly Alzheimer's disease, although scientists are working hard on this. Due to the fact that BA protein has multiple roles, there will be multiple causes of the illness, which makes us believe that there will never be a single effective treatment for which we will set forth a bold and revolutionary new paradigm for the disease to be addressed.

The paradigm of approaching the treatment of Alzheimer's disease:

The approach on preventing or treating Alzheimer's dementia should be centred on the patient. A rigorous casuistic classification of Alzheimer's dementia is required. Then depending on the category, the treatment will be applied accordingly.

You see dear readers, the importance of such approaching is due to a multitude of reasons that cause dementia. Here, we will add that a disorder in functionality at mitochondrial level as well can be linked with certain diseases like epilepsy, stroke, bipolar disorder, chronic fatigue syndrome, schizophrenia Parkinson etc. and dementia Alzheimer's disease **(Lim YA, Rhein V, Baysang G, Meier F, Poljak A, Raftery MJ, Guilhaus M, Ittner LM, Eckert A, Götz J (April 2010). 'Abeta and human amylin share a common toxicity pathway via mitochondrial dysfunction.' Proteomics. 10 (8): 1621–33)**. Mitochondria is converting energy for cell respiration. It takes the oxygen from the lungs to oxidise the glucose, and this way, providing further the necessary energy for the cell, and if something goes wrong in this process, it may lead to Alzheimer's disease as well. For instance, if there is a leakage of activated oxygen from the mitochondria during oxidative phosphorylation, may occur oxidative stress which, in this case, a super production of beta-amyloid may be triggered because as we have shown previously this multi-functional protein plays an important role in protection against oxidative stress as well. To make it a little easier for the readers, oxidative stress is caused by the imbalance between reactive oxygen production and the capacity of biological system to detoxify rapidly or repair from the resulted damage. So you see dear readers, there are more reasons as well for the presence of beta-amyloid in large quantities in the brain. That's why in order to heal or treat properly a patient with Alzheimer's disease, it is very important to know the exact cause.

2.2 Brain Shrinking Does Not Necessarily Cause Dementia.

In order to achieve one of the goals proposed in this work, we return to what was said previously regarding the relationship between brain shrinking and dementia: *not dementia causes brain shrinking, but shrinking of the brain can lead to dementia, and this only under certain circumstances. The location where the first atrophy of the brain will occur, early symptoms may be revealed. These symptoms are different from each other due to the fact that different parts of the brain are affected provided that each part of the brain has its own function which may be manifested trough behaviour.*

Demonstration of this idea requires us a return in time, mainly in 1871, when one of the greatest revolutionaries of science, the great Charles Darwin (1809–1882) observed among other things, that rabbits kept living in a small cage, have up to 15–30% brain shrinkage comparative to those who live and develop freely in nature.

How does this explain? Well, the environmental challenges make the individuals to develop their neural capacity through formation of new synapses by learning from new experiences. While the individual in a restricted environment, such as the rabbit in a cage, is only being offered a very small number of challenges, the learning of new experiences is drastically reduced so that neurogenesis will not be stimulated too much either. From here, we conclude that a person whose average number of active neuronal synapses larger is than that of a person with lower average active synapses may have a different neurogenesis rate.

In people happens according to the same principle; for instance, neglected children, in their early development, have a less developed brain in volume, especially the prefrontal cortex than those who have affection, care and education.

In the case of adopted orphaned children, the same thing happens, those adopted up to the age of two will generally exceed an IQ of 100, while those adopted between the ages of 2–6 will have an IQ of about 80 **(D Swaab, 2010)**.

We will present a case study of a patient of American psychiatrist Bruce Perry in 1995.

A two-month-old boy was left permanently in the care of his grandmother by his 15-year-old mother when he was born. His grandmother could only take care of him until he was 11 months old because suffering from an illness, she passed away, so her boyfriend got to take further care of the baby. Being over 60 years of age, things were pretty tough raising the baby on his own, so he got in touch with Child Protection Services to relocate the baby to another family. The people from this organisation said that they were going to look for a good family for the boy, but it would take some time, and the man seeming to be okay to them, agreed the baby to stay with him until a new family will be found to adopt the little one.

Having receiving no news from this organisation, the child remained with him. Being a dog breeder, the man had put the child in a cage…not knowing what else to do with this little human!

This child was raised up to six years old in this cage, with only water, food and clean nappies, his name was Justin. During all this time, he was very rarely spoken to; he was totally deprived of any kind of affection, no one was playing with him either.

At the age of two, he was taken to the hospital by his caregiver because he did not speak, did not walk and had severe signs of mental retardation which gave him the diagnosis of static encephalopathy which means severe cerebral diseases of unknown origin with minimal probabilities of recovery.

Many tests, including an MRI scan, have been done on this occasion, and it has been found that the boy presented a decrease in size of cerebral cortex similar to that of an Alzheimer's patient. The circumference of his head was as small as a one-year-old child.

To be noted the fact that nobody at the hospital asked anything about the environment in which this child grows and develops!

Actually, by chance, a pneumonia made it happened for the boy to get to Texas Children's Hospital when he was six years old…and this way, saved his life living as an animal at his former caretaker. There the child's behaviour was limited to screaming, throwing faeces and foods at the caregivers, especially since his new location resembled to a cage being actually a special place for dangerous patients. Even only for a sanguine analysis was needed force to hold him down for taking blood samples.

Then was called at the paediatric intensive care unit of the hospital to doctor Bruce Perry. He spoke to the child's caretaker Arthur, revealing that for the first time he was speaking about the 'home' situation of the child, for the simple reason that nobody ever asked him anything about it.

A few months later, the child making great progress in his development, such as bipedal walking, word learning, and appropriate communication, was placed in a family with a supportive development environment for this child. At the age of eight, he was enrolled at the kindergarten in the four-year-old group.

Similar cases are known as well, of which we mention the case of a feral child (wolf child) named 'Victor' by the famous French doctor Jean Marc Gaspard Itard from 1797. This child was living in the woods completely isolated from outside world before he was captured. By that time he was around 12 years old. After that, he was given various caretakers from which he escaped eight times before doctor Itard took him in his own house. Although Victor made progress in behaviour towards other people and language understanding, he could never got to speak properly because we believe it is a matter of major underdevelopment of the brain in specific language areas called Broca en Wernicke, respectively, due to an absolute solitary life, away from humans, where language stimulation was almost nil during his first 12 years of his life. To make it a little easier for our readers, area Broca is predominantly involved in speaking the language and Wernicke area in understanding the language, so if those areas are underdeveloped as in Victor's case, serious problems will occur at communication level. It is also important to mention that language acquirements are best made before the age of 12. That explains the phenomenon why children acquire a foreign language faster, easier and accentless than their parents if they spend the same amount of time or immigrating to a foreign country.

Another case we wish to bring to our readers attention is the experiment of Emperor Frederick II von Hohenstaufen of Holy Roman Empire in thirteen century that tried to discover the language of God or so-called Hebrew considered at the time the first language on earth because he believed it would have been revealed if one did not learn his mother tongue, so by kidnapping a dozens of children before they could learn to speak and keeping them together in isolation, they will instantly begin to communicate among each other by speaking in Hebrew or Greek, Latin, Arabic or the tongue of their parents at once. The boys were washed and fed by foster mothers and that was about it because they were not allowed to talk to them. Well...the boys did not live for too long because they were living in complete isolation and none of them ever got to speak in any proper language just trough gestures, some sounds, showing emotions, clapping hands and blandishments, so the experiment was a total failure. This experiment was recorded by an Italian monk called Salimbene di Adam (1221–1290) in his work Cronica (Chronicles). We do not know for certain if Frederick was inspired by the Egyptian Pharaoh Psammetichus the first (664–610 BC) who did rather a similar experiment on languages that lead him to the conclusion that the capacity of speech is innate, and the natural language of human beings is Phrygian because after two years, the word 'becos' came up from the mouth of the boys who he was experimenting upon. Becos in Phrygian meant bread...This word is probably the precursor of baking in English, baken in Dutch or backen in German. Well, Pharaoh Psammetichus was half closed to the truth with his observations made around 2600 years ago. The capacity of speech is, indeed, innate since we are, genetically, equipped with all the mechanisms required for this form of communication, but this does not mean we are born with a spoken language. A language is acquired by a learning process and not being born with it. Although very interesting, we have to leave the field of linguistics and return to our topics before we get carried away from our main subject.

So after all the above described cases, we came to a bunch of conclusions, mainly, isolation at young age leads to underdevelopment in size of the brain as whole, in language areas of the cerebral cortex, and the subjects that are dying young...of course, implicitly major behaviour problems due to lack of affection as a result of isolation.

Through all of these above cases, we infer that drastic reduction of the brain in size is not only due to environmental factors, but also age and as well as a result of a genetical deviation regarding morphological aspect of the brain; therefore, *shrinking of the brain is not a determining factor in the aetiology of dementia.*

Regarding the reduction of cerebral cortex volume in Alzheimer's disease, we can say that it is due to a drastic reduction in size of key components of the central nervous system due to their deterioration such as hippocampus, thalamic structures, parietal cortex temporal cortex etc. which extend from one to the other.

In other order of ideas, *not the shrinking of the brain itself leads by definition to dementia, but the functional impairment of one or more parts of the brain determines this matter.*

In the case of Alzheimer's disease, besides the fact that due to aging, the brain already suffers a natural decrease in volume, there is on top of that an accelerated erosion of the cerebral cortex and its internal structures as well.

This possible accelerated erosion is primarily due to beta-amyloid protein presence in large quantities, and this way becoming toxic for the brain. Due to the sticky nature of this protein, it will deposit in so-called senile plaques and, therein, lies the toxicity of beta-amyloid. Here, it is important to add the possible factor of a malfunctioning recycling circulation of the cerebrospinal fluid from the cranial cavity for some reason. It is of a paramount importance that removal of cleaning waste from the brain to be done properly by the cerebrospinal fluid system.

Fluid movement in the brain is pulsatile and determined by the heartbeat, so any anomaly at this level (low heartbeat and blood pressure) will influence at certain extent proper cleansing of the brain waste which, of course, contains beta-amyloid plaques as well among other things. In this case, the complete refreshing cycle every four hours, as we have mentioned, will be like three or two or even less times a day which on the long run inevitably the concentration of beta-amyloid plaques will get higher.

We said possible accelerated erosion because the cleaning system of the cell residues in brain can operate very well but what if it cannot cope with too much beta-amyloid flow? It would be very important to know how long does it take before the BA protein starts to deposit in plaques.

According to the foregoing, the highest concentration of both the hyperphosphorylated Tau protein and the presenile plaques of beta-amyloid are in the hippocampus. The beta-amyloid protein is produced by the hippocampal structures and the largest plaques density is there as well, which means that its deposition in plaques occurs very quickly, which exceeds the recycling capacity of the circulatory system of the cerebrospinal fluid in that area.

Also, in the hippocampus is the highest concentration of microglia attacking these BA plaques or plates but in the same time as well the healthy tissue of the brain cells in this region which leads to carvings in this highly important part of the brain as we have described previously.

Analogue happens in the cerebral cortex where, according to the above principle, the bottoms of the circumvolutions are widening and deepening as a result of erosions at the base of their walls. The circumvolution is the portion of the cerebral cortex between two brain ditches.

By deduction, we can say that this form of dementia is actually a disease of the whole body drastically affecting the hippocampus because this area is mostly damaged according to studies that clearly show a morphological difference of this part of the brain compared to other forms of dementia.

In conclusion, we can say by the above shown that reduction of cerebral cortex in size is not determinant in dementia but is a consequence of cellular activities within the central nervous system in response to external environmental factors, genetic factors or a combination of these.

2.3 A Brief Incursion on Symptomatology of Alzheimer's Disease

Before displaying our ideas in this new subchapter, we need first to answer the following question: ***When is it dementia?*** Because every one of us happened to go to either the kitchen or the next room forgetting why we went there in first place, each one of us happened to have a lapsus or to forget the name of a thing, especially if is not often used or to forget where we put certain things…There are a lot of reasons why such things can happen to us without being diagnosed with some kind of dementia.

But if we go shopping and we do not know what we're doing there, or we often forget the names of the things we frequently use, if we forget the past or who are the closest persons to us or we do not know how to anoint a slice of bread anymore etc., then the problem becomes clear.

Factors that cause forgetting as a temporary phenomenon are many of which we mentioned the most common ones:

- Older age, brain functions no longer work on the youth parameters.
- Traumatic injuries at head level following to certain blows to that area.
- Some drug treatments such as long-term use of sleeping pills, various hormonal treatments with testosterone or other endocrine treatments, narcosis.
- Diet, a deficiency of vitamins can affect the supply of energy cells such as vitamin B found in meat plays a very important role here. Let's not forget that a

reduction of water in the body also produces forgetfulness and attention disturbances at some point. Abuse of alcohol can cause memory disorders or even Korsakov dementia.

- Various infectious or thyroid diseases.
- Various chemical environment such carbon monoxide.
- Worries affects attention, concentration and, therefore, frequent occurrence of forgetfulness.
- Low interest on certain topics makes the attention to be very low, and this way retaining the information is considerably diminished, which will prevent the remembrance of those things related from the topics (a phenomenon very often encountered in schools among the pupils due to personal reasons or not so good didactic skills of the teacher).
- Tiredness and especially sleep deprivations which even after a one night without sleep higher accumulation of beta-amyloid are registered in the brain according to the newest studies of University of California.

Forgetfulness, sometimes, causes some inconveniences, but it does not affect everyday life, but a sufferer of dementia, regardless of its type, not only has daily problems, but the people around are affected by its illness as well.

For a better understanding, we offer a few examples of memory disorders in healthy persons and ill with Alzheimer's disease:

Healthy person:

- Forgetting the details; for example, who was at your birthday party a couple of years ago.
- A name or designation of a thing that is on the 'tip of the tongue' when someone tells you, immediately is reminded.

- Retrieving new information is a little bit more difficult, sometimes, and costs a higher concentration but is still working.

Person ill with Alzheimer's disease:

- Forgetting the whole event; for example, own birthday which took place with a little while ago.
- The impression that information has disappeared from memory, a name or a designation cannot be remembered (recognised) even if someone else is saying it still does not mean a thing to them
- The learning capacity is affected, the new information received is almost not retained at all.
- Forgetting the names of their children or spouses or being even not able to recognise them at all.
- Not being able to remember how to anoint a slice of bread.

Dementia is characterised by progressive degenerative advancement of the cognitive and, finally, physiological functions of the sufferer. So we can say that the symptoms of Alzheimer's disease are divided into two categories, namely the psychopathological and physiological symptomatology.

We will present the two categories of symptoms below, and we will begin with cognitive signs of Alzheimer's dementia.

Psychopathological symptoms

- ### _Forgetfulness_
The sufferer forgets the new information, the place and date of important events. They often ask the same questions and become dependent of to do lists…if they remember they have a list of these things. Hygiene because the sufferer forgets to take care of it.

- ***Problems with usual things***

Normal things, for example, making a basic financial situation or taking care of certain hobbies become very difficult as well.

- ***Spatial and time confusions***

Appreciation of time becomes increasingly cumbersome as a result of which the sufferer cannot pronounce itself only with great difficulty upon a representation in the form of drawing a given date like what time is it. The patient has trouble remembering what day of the week it is, in which month, season or year. Orientation in space also becomes difficult because it no longer recognises the places; for instance, it does not know anymore where the bathroom is in their own house. Wandering on the streets at night occur at a certain point.

- ***Language***

Indicates that the temporal cortex area is affected more specifically area Broca, Wernicke's or even both. The use and understanding of language becomes very difficult for Alzheimer's sufferers; therefore, they have problems to follow a conversation, the meaning of simple words is forgotten, deformation of writing suggesting that the fine motor area is affected at the level of basal ganglia. More and more serious problems occur in remembering the names of things. Severe loss of communication capabilities will later occur.

- ***The loss of things***

The sufferer forgets where he puts things, and these are often in very unlikely places such as the wallet in the fridge, the keys in the letterbox etc.

- ***Estimative capacity loss***

Situational estimation becomes very cumbersome for which decision-making capacity is also compromised. Persons suffering from dementia can no longer appreciate; for example, how much is a discount in price, they often buy things that are not necessary and spend large sums of money. Sometimes, they keep buying things all over again because they forgot they bought that before.

- ### *Social isolation*
Due to the fact that Alzheimer's sufferers are aware at first of the problems they face due to the disease, they begin to self-isolate in order to not to embarrass themselves in front of other people; they retire, for example, watching programs on TV or sleeping very often, things that are proven to be very bad for any person on the long-term.

Also, it is very important to mention here the researches of the neuropsychologist Uysal-Bozkir on older migrant people that in the sixties came to the Netherlands as guest workers, where dementia rate is 3–4 times higher than their Dutch counterparts of the same age level. This group of foreigners are suffering from loneliness and show depressive symptoms as well which on the long-term may lead to dementia **(De Volkskrant Sept. 2016)**. So you see how important social life can be…Depression can be one of the first symptoms of Alzheimer's disease according to some of the famous specialists, but we have to specify the fact that depression can lead to dementia as well. So depression can be a symptom of an illness but also the main cause of an illness. So this idea clearly reflects and explains the difference between the medical paradigms of the ancient Egyptians and Thracians mentioned early in this work. That is also one of the reasons why depression is considered in certain countries a disease and in some countries not.

- ### *Changes in behaviour and personality*
One of the first symptoms of Alzheimer's disease is episodic disorders at empathy level. Emotional values can no longer be controlled and assigned to new things in order to retain them in memory.

Persons suffering from dementia are becoming confused, suspicious, depressed, fearful and, without any specific reason, can become aggressive and even resorting to violence.

- ### *States of agitation*

It seems that a dementia sufferer is excessively looking for something, sometimes, usually not knowing why, or wants to clean where already it's been cleaned, or has to do something but does not know what exactly. This state of unrest is affecting sleeping, thus, favouring the overproduction of beta-amyloid protein leading to considerable increase of presenile plaques.

- ### *Perceptual problems*

Sufferers of Alzheimer's present difficulties in assessing the distance, colour or contrast difference although their eyes are working well; they no longer recognise themselves in the mirror and start to communicate with their own reflection, hallucinations depending on their inner emotions; they can see snakes, mice, people long ago deceased, angels etc. As it advances, occurs a fragmentation of spatial and temporal perception. Old memories become more and more vivid. Past events come more often in the mind, and it is possible to confuse the present and the past.

People from the past are perceived in present and those present are not recognised or seen at present.

As the disease progresses, physiological problems will occur from which we mention the most important below:

Physiological symptoms

- Chewing Food, the patient loses the ability to chew, which leads to the occurrence of digestive problems.
- Motoric difficulties in lower limbs, thus, appearing steady walking problems.
- Bladder infections due to lack of physical exercise.
- Loss of ability to control the mechanisms of removing toxins from the body (urinary and faecal incontinency).

- Functionality problems at the respiratory system level.

Alzheimer's dementia is an infernal illness that drastically influences the life and behaviour of the individual as well as for the people around like family members or friends care givers. Here, we can say that psychological help for the patient is only useful at the beginning because later on when the forgetfulness episodes will occur…it is not much a psychologist can do anymore.

Alzheimer's disease cannot be cured yet, but there are treatments to relieve some of the symptoms…unfortunately, this is all what the therapy can offer for dementia sufferers right now.

It is necessary to pay special attention to the caregiver of the patient, and here, we do not refer to specialised staff from institutionalisation centres, but to a close relative or friend of the sufferer, usually a member of the family.

The caregiver, however, feels the greatest pressure at a certain point in the intermediary phase of the illness when the patient loses his independence, needs to be given special attention, so instead, the psychologist have to concentrate on the caregivers. The impact on this person is enormous, especially when it has to respond to the patient's needs 24/7 on a stretch that lasts over a few years! The stress accumulated by the caretaker during this time can drastically affect his health, even long after the patient has gone into the world of non-existence. We should not forget that under stressful conditions, the adrenal glands will produce large amounts of cortisol which in the long run will shorten considerably its life. Cortisol in the short-term is beneficial but on the long-term becomes a killer, thus, affecting the whole neuroendocrine system of the body. For society, it is enough to lose one of its members because of Alzheimer's disease, so it is necessary to give all necessary support to the caregiver, not to lose another one because of a physical and emotional degradation due to given care. Those people need to have special care from the psychologists, they have to be mentally strong enough to cope with the responsibility of the patient on the long run. It is of a paramount importance that care-giving people should be feeling that they are supported adequately by the psychologists, and they should never feel left alone by those specialists. Inadequate psychological help offered by the specialists will negatively influence the state of mind of the caregiver and implicitly on the quality of the care received by the patient or worse.

As we mentioned above, for various reasons, a sufferer does not always have somebody around like a close relative or a friend. In this case, the patient needs to be institutionalised in specialised clinics where he is treated and supported by specialised personnel. There, too, the psychologists have to give special care to those people even though they are trained to help the patients. It is of a paramount importance that a caregiver should not hesitate to ask for any help if feels things are getting too much for them at a certain point.

As we have shown in the previous chapter that Alzheimer's disease begins 20 years before it is manifested or even present since birth, we cannot talk about dementia at that point.

Dementia, especially in the early symptomatic phase, can only be declared in relation with symptomatic manifestations and after confirmation of the analyses and tests done by the specialists in the field...so after a scientific understanding of the phenomenon.

Usually, Alzheimer's sufferers are accompanied when they go to a doctor by either a close relative or a friend. Companions are actually those providing first-hand information on the condition of the suffering person to the specialised staff. In some cases, this illness is discovered accidentally with the MRI scan when checking different problems like concussions for instance.

"The word pain does not begin to mean anything other than the moment when it reminds us of a sensation that we have already experienced."

– Denis Diderot

Chapter III. Hippocampus and Amygdala, the Informational Traffic Node

3.1 Hippocampus

We start this chapter with the wisdom words of the great French thinker Denis Diderot (1713–1784) in which he actually speaks of pain but contains exactly what we are interested in, mainly, the principle of memory function in relation to a given fact.

In this case, the given fact is the pain itself which is nothing but a sensation perceived by the sensory systems, further analysed and interpreted in order to react accordingly.

Sensation is the first mental level of processing, interpreting and using an information about the attributes of objects and phenomena of the external environment, and about the inner state of the body. It is the primary source of knowledge. Other than through sensations, we cannot get any data about things and surrounding phenomena **(M Golu, 2007)**.

There is nothing in the intellect that previously did not exist in the senses – *Nihil est in intelectum quo prior non fuerit in sensum* **(John Locke)**.

Well, the information but also the reactions to them are retained by memory through the principle of comparison.

First, it is very important to know the role of emotions which is to produce a specific response to a stimulus. Emotions are mental and bodily responses that are deployed automatically when an organism recognises that a situation warrants such a reaction **(Damasio, 1994)**.

Schematically, a sensation is retained in memory when given an emotional value by the structures of the limbic and reptilian systems according to its intensity. A new sensation of the same type is compared by the intensity of its emotional value to the previous sensation where according to that will be reacting upon in one way or another.

It should be specified that to any stimulus is attributed an emotional value in order to be retained in memory, but it is different from individual to individual due to the different sensitivity of each person's senses based on individual sensory and inner experiences.

The emotional value that is awaken by an object lies in a sensory-emotional range comprised in a pleasant and unpleasant scale. **Why?** Because the strongest emotions are produced by horror (fear of high intensity) and ecstasy (high intensity of pleasure).

These are the standard emotional values of instincts in the limbic system and reptilian brain, and any emotional value of a stimulus is between these two extremities. These are part of the survival systems that interact with environmental stimuli through the senses.

The response to a given stimulus has in principle another emotional load sometimes than the stimulus inspired by it, given the fact that is processed by the cognitive structures of neocortex which we call reactive emotional load according to the data collected by the senses about that stimulus based on distance, for instance, or the emotional set of the individual at that given moment because in accordance with it changes the intensity of a reaction. Hippocampus, this is the part of the brain that makes the connection between emotion and location memory. Also, we have to mention the fact that, sometimes, the emotional intensity reaches high values that trigger the actions from the reptilian brain (basal ganglia nodes) the so-called fight, flight or freeze mode. How this principle work is very thorough described in the book *Essay on the classification of human traditional senses* by the same author of this present work.

We can distinguish two forms of emotional load, they are:

- *Instinctive emotional load – limbic system (amygdala) – reptilian brain (basal ganglia, cerebellum and brainstem)*
- *Cognitive emotional load – neocortex*

By what we have said so far, we can say that it is an input/output system of the emotions awakened by the stimulus (input) and the emotional load of the response or reaction (output).

The functionality of this emotional input/output system is possible due to the continuous tandem of the three systems, namely neocortical, limbic and reptilian.

We consider it necessary to make a brief description of the human brain based on the theory of American physician **Paul D MacLean**.

According to the author of this revolutionary theory, the brain along the evolution of the human species is formed from three distinct parts, namely the reptilian complex, the limbic system and the neocortex.

Here we have to make the following statement, all three brain formations are also found in reptiles, but the most developed part of their brain is the basal ganglia or reptilian complex as MacLean called it. At the same time, these brain formations are interconnected with each other, so that the reptilian side is permanently connected to the limbic system and neocortex.

From the anthropo-physical evolutionary point of view, the reptilian and limbic brain did not suffer significant morphological changes in volume, but instead, the neocortex is the one with major volumetric significance compared to our ancestors who had less developed brain in size.

Reptilian brain

The reptilian brain is at the base of the so-called telencephalic brain and is responsible for instinctive thinking, voluntary motor movements, balancing, learning, routine formation, eye movements, and last but not least, cognition (instinct) and emotions.

So for example, if we are caught by surprise by a high-intensity sound in our immediate vicinity, the auditory senses will trigger the imminent alarm signal, and the reptilian brain immediately inject a huge flow of GABA neurotransmitters to temporarily inhibit the activity of neocortex and rational thinking. **Why?** Just because the basal ganglia knows that the neocortex reaction rate is, at least, twice as low, and so the body is exposed to danger for a longer period of time. That's why the decision will be summed up to one of the three instinctual responses, namely: *fighting, freezing or fleeing.*

Neocortical thinking plans, analyses the number of variants and this costs time, or it is particularly vital in imminent danger situations. Let us not forget that we are talking about circumstances in which an immediate reaction, one of the three is required namely, freezing, fleeing or fighting where there is no planning because there is not enough time for that.

Please note that the basal ganglia is using predominantly neurotransmitters GABA, which are inhibitors but that does not mean that it uses only these. So when the basal ganglia suppresses rational thinking in the neocortex they also trigger adrenal glands that produce a massive adrenaline flow necessary to set the body in one of the stages of fighting, freezing or fleeing.

Neocortex

Neocortex is the most developed area of the human brain. It is responsible for cognitive functions such as sensory perception, motor control, sense of spatial orientation, feeling of emotions, movement of arms and legs and language.

This is where the neocortical thinking or reasoning occurs, while neocortex sends sensory information or rational-type movements to the reptilian brain. Finally, the reptilian brain, in turn, sends the instinctual decisions back to the neocortex for the answer. All information exchange between neocortex and reptilian brain is passed through limbic system.

Limbic system

Limbic system or the emotional brain is located between neocortex and reptilian brain and is responsible for processing and regulating emotions, memory, sexual activities etc. Here is also the neuroendocrine system of the central nervous system as well as the processing of information obtained by the olfactory perceptual organs. The limbic system is linked to the basal ganglia at the level of thalamic structures.

Thalamus plays a particularly important role in perception, attention, alert, consciousness, sleep, timing and movement. Limbic system connects many parts of the brain to each other, which is extremely important, here is the junction of information coming from different areas of the brain.

Here, we deduce the role of dispatcher of the received information from a region of the brain and directed to others via the *hippocampus.*

Hippocampus means seahorse in Greek due to the striking shape similarity with these tiny sea creatures. Mammals and humans have two of these structures and are actually called *hippocampi* together. They are symmetrically disposed in each of the two cerebral hemispheres and are not functional identical. Experiments done on mice showed a left-right functional dissociation in hippocampal memory performance.

Hippocampi are part of the limbic system and play a particularly important role in the junctions between short memory and long memory, in spatial orientation, and we add is the *information traffic junction or node*, when it comes to memory formation but that does not mean that memory stacks in the hippocampus because this is stored in the cerebral cortex.

Schematically, an information obtained through our senses is taken temporarily by neuron formations from the related part of neocortex and brought to hippocampus, and from there, this information, after is loaded with a certain emotional value, is sent back to cerebral cortex where it will become a long-term memory kind of information. Hippocampus has its own memory only to ensure the proper functioning of information traffic between the six brain areas. These areas are:

- ***Frontal lobe***
- ***Temporal lobe***
- ***Parietal lobe***
- ***Occipital lobe***
- ***Cerebellum***
- ***Brainstem***

We emphasise that at the level of memory, hippocampus ensures the junction between various parts of the brain's memories. These are specific memories according to senses they represent.

Through hippocampus passes input and output information, each of which is specific information so that their traffic is made via the appropriate hippocampal lobe. In other words, ***the information input enters through a lobe and information output comes out through the other lobe.*** But that is not strictly so because if one of the hippocampal lobes are removed, the remaining one will take over the functions of the extracted one and both input and output information will go through the remaining lobe. However, patients with a right hippocampal lobe removed will experience either problems with short memory or long memory. But if whole hippocampus will be removed, long-term memory consolidation would not be possible. Certain types of memory are still functional even in those circumstances because they are using different pathways for different memories in the brain as well. Here, we take the freedom to bring to our readers' attention the most studied case in the world regarding hippocampus removal from 1953 of a young man named Henry Molaison. After an accident, his skull got badly cracked, and after that, it occurred to this individual severe seizures and a surgery had to be performed in which the whole hippocampus had to be removed.

Although the operation had been successfully regarded because the seizures no longer occurred, his personality remained intact, and even his IQ had improved, the patient's memory, however, was shot. He lost most of his memory from his previous decade...He was 27 at that time, was unable to form new memories, forgetting what day it was, repeated comments, eating multiple meals in a row; therefore, somebody had to stop him from that; otherwise, he will eat to death; he was watching old movies over and over and were still new to him because he could not remember what he already watch many times before.

Human brain uses different kind of memories assigned by different parts of the brain that are involved in emotions such as amygdala, basal ganglia, brainstem, cerebellum, hypothalamus so because some of those areas were still intact and could interact among each other even without hippocampus, Henry Molaison could have a functional life up to a certain extent without inability to form new memory.

In our view, we tend to believe that the intermediate emotional load given to input and output information is given by the immediate vicinity of the hippocampus, namely the *amygdala*, but it is not the only one because basal ganglia, brainstem hypothalamus and cerebellum play an important role on this matter as well.

3.2 Amygdala

Amygdala, better known as the amygdalae, because they are two of them, is the almond-shaped parts that rests on the hippocampus. Like the latter, it consists of two lobes, each of which has distinct roles. It plays a very important role in the processing of memory and emotions, decision-making and emotional responses. This structure also plays a key role modulating memory for emotional context **(Rudy, Huff & Matus-Amat, 2004; Malin & McGaugh, 2006)**.

It is part of the limbic system and is also considered part of the basal ganglia nodes. The amygdala has connections to multiple parts of the brain such as the olfactory cortex, the orbital and medial structures of the prefrontal cortex, and is in, particularly, close connection to thalamic, hippocampal and sensory structures. Also, recent research suggests that the amygdalae are, in fact, structurally **(Szabo et al., 2001)** and functionally asymmetrical **(see Baas, Aleman, & Kahn, 2004; Zald, 2003)**. Just like the hippocampus.

A particularly important thing has been published in the US National Library of Medicine by Finnish researchers at the Institute of Molecular Sciences at Kuopio University in Finland regarding the fact that *the most consistent reciprocity of the connections between amygdala and hippocampus structures is in the entorhinal cortex area!!!* **(A Pitkanen, M Pikkarainen, N Nurminen, A Ylinen, 2000)**.

This publication of Finnish researchers supports the hypothesis that we are trying to show that in Alzheimer's dementia, memory is not lost in its entirety but cannot be accessed, which is observed from the episodic remembrance phenomena of the patients.

To explain the phenomenon, we return to the fact that to any stimulus or to any information is assigned an emotional load by one of the parts of amygdala, basal ganglia, cerebellum and brainstem as well in order to be retained in memory, and, therefore, to be able to be recognised in order to further response that needs to be given through its emotional load by the other side.

The stimulus or an emotionally loaded information by one of the amygdala will be transmitted further through the hippocampal structures of the same corresponding part at the entorhinal cortex level. Analogous for the response case. We remind our readers that in Alzheimer's disease the entorhinal cortex is the most affected cerebral region. So the progressive failure of the memory access mechanisms (memory recollection) is directly due to extent of damage of this area called enthorhinal corthex. The mnesic awakenings or the episodical recollection of memory is occurring due to a temporary revitalisation of the enthorhinal corthex triggered by a crucial improvement of a certain body condition.

The informational input received by the amygdala is done through the sensory systems of the senses. It is sent through the hippocampus to the specific region containing the corresponding memory of the sense or senses underlying the collection of information about a given stimulus.

Once this specific memory is accessed, it is emotionally loaded by the amygdala for the contextual response processed by neocortex. Here, we have to specify something very important, not every stimulus is emotionally loaded by amygdala only the specific ones. Therefore, we will refer to the case of SM, a lady whose both amygdalae were surgically extracted and lost her ability of fear. The nature of fear is survival and the amygdala helps us stay alive by avoiding situations, people or objects that put our life in danger. So the amygdala is analysing the potential of a danger. Because SM is missing her amygdala, she is also missing the ability to detect and avoid danger in the world. "It is quite remarkable that she is still alive," said Justin Feinstein of the University of Iowa. However, she was not absolutely fear-proof because experiments shown the presence of a great deal of high intensity fear and panic attacks when she experienced suffocation with carbon dioxide, and the feeling she got was completely new to her.

That got all scientist off guard as well. *How is it possible to still experience fear without amygdalae?* Well…our explanation is that once the extraction of amygdalae was performed, the mechanisms of emotional loading of specific stimuli were removed, too. So the brain did not perceive the danger that normally should be expressed by physical stimuli in certain circumstances at the level of basal ganglia and set the body for fight, freeze and flee mode for not being able to receive the input from the amygdala because it was removed. However, when SM experienced suffocation with carbon dioxide, she did feel fear, but that was due to *brain stem* and *hypothalamus*. The later, regulates thirst, response to pain, levels of pleasure, sexual satisfaction, anger and aggressive behaviour, autonomic control, sleep and wakefulness, endocrine control body temperature. Also, neurons controlling cardiovascular responses to emotion are located in lateral hypothalamus-perifornical region **(OA Smith, JL DeVito and CA Astley, 1990)**.

Brain stem regulates the functioning of the *autonomic nervous system*, which, in turn, means it regulates things like pulse, blood pressure, *breathing*, temperature, sleep and wakefulness and arousal in response to emotional circumstances, reflexes for sneezing, vomiting and coughing. In conclusion, the fear of suffocation which is an emotion was triggered by the brain stem and further by the hypothalamus. Feelings or sensations, our perceptions of what is going on around us, define which emotions are created **(Wolfe, 2010)**. Our amygdala creates the feelings, and the hypothalamus creates emotions from those feelings **(Britannica, 2008; Wolfe, 2010)**. Here, we find important to mention than not only amygdala creates the feelings but only the specific ones because other brain parts involved in emotions are doing that as well and they all cross the hippocampus.

We must emphasise that to the same stimulus can be given different emotional value loads depending on the subject's perception corroborated with inner state of mind at a given moment.

This principle underlies the diversified utility to the same stimulus. It can now be argued that this is due to creativity, but we must not forget that creativity itself would not have been possible without the emotions that underlie any representations. This explains that in the case of Alzheimer's disease, the learning process is affected precisely due to the deterioration of emotional capacities and, therefore, certain memories cannot be accessed and/or formed.

In other words, the stimulus information is no longer properly loaded with the associated emotional values to be accordingly recognised by cognitive functions.

Now comes the question of *why a certain stimulus is no longer properly loaded with emotional value?*

To answer this question, we refer to one of the features of Alzheimer's disease, namely the hippocampal structures, more precisely, of the entorhinal cortex as the most affected part of the brain in this disease.

In the entorhinal cortex, among other things, the most intense communication between the amygdala and the hippocampus takes place, and, therefore, the emotional value-attributable system of the amygdala is affected, where these structures are simply 'eaten' by Alzheimer's disease.

Volume and hence morphological changes of the hippocampus and amygdala are recorded even due to depression or even in conditions of continuous anxiety. High cortisol streams emitted under stress conditions attack the hippocampus, thus, reducing it to as much as 80% of the volume so that neurogenesis is drastically impaired **(R Kahn 2006)**. From here, we can deduce a new possibility that causes memory sequentially to come and go to an Alzheimer's patient as being related to hippocampal size. When this brain structure reaches a critical decrease point in size memory will get severely impaired, and the patient will not recognise its own family for instance.

Analogously when hippocampus increases in size to a point where the patient is recognising its family again. Perhaps if we know the reason of increasing in size of the hippocampus and master it than the key towards healing will be in our hands. We believe if we are eliminating as much as possible the things that are bad for us from stress, nutrition etc. and increase the amount of good things from stress (positive), nutrition, physical exercise, passion for things etc., will modify the size of hippocampus. More research on this matter needs to be performed.

Alzheimer's sufferer, as we have previously argued, has moments when it remembers things, feelings, loved ones and so on, proves that memory has not disappeared; otherwise, the patient would not have had the opportunity to remember them. Memory is present all the time, but accessing it by the brain is only allowed episodically under circumstances unknown yet.

Here, we are taking the freedom to reveal to our readers, the case of Kelly Gunderson's mother, an 87-year-old lady who was suffering from Alzheimer's disease. This elderly woman did not recognise her daughter long before one day when the two of them were conversing as usual, the mother answered affirmatively to her daughter's question if she knew who she was even naming her name while minutes before she did not recognised her at all as her own daughter *(the movie is on YouTube even posted by Kelly Gunderson in 2014)*.

From the reactions point of view, the mother had a natural reaction without a special joy, but a very normal behaviour when she remembered, but her daughter, instead, had a startling surprise.

From here, we deduce that for the patient, the period when memory was not accessed was not significant but, in return, for Kelly was because she responded surprised and happy in the same time.

Another very important thing we've noticed is when Kelly asked her mom what was she thinking at before, when asking her if she knew her, and she was answering it with 'no' that she does not know her who she is. Then her mother responded that she did not know what she was thinking of.

This is explained by the fact that her daughter Kelly did not get recognised who she might be to her mother in moments of non-recognition because the stimulus in person of her daughter Kelly was not loaded with adequate emotional value, and so it did not ring any bell to the patient about the person who was talking to her. She had no idea who her daughter was.

At the same time, it is remarked the very interesting fact that the patient remembered the moment when she did not recognise Kelly, which means that memory recorded those moments. Was not like…what are you talking about, I have always recognised you! But she did remember not recognising her daughter. So something triggered her memory…but what? Whatever it might have been, it was happening in the hippocampus – amygdala formations in the emotional value-attributable system…but it could be something else as well like an adrenalin rush.

Such cases of patients who are temporarily 'recovering' memory are many but noteworthy is that when they are in the terminal phase and death begins to smile at them, they give signs of mnesic awakening' as we can call it such, as reported by the caregiver staff of a geriatric clinic in the Netherlands. Some of the patients are starting to talk normally in one go even after a long period of vegetability fact that stuns everybody around.

We can say that patients, somehow, feel the fear of death. It is not yet known the principle after which memory is accessed again in the last act of their life. We suppose that fear, which is the most powerful emotion, causes adrenaline to be triggered in the body, and this, in turn, causes 'mnesic awakenings' recollecting the memory.

One of the characteristics of adrenaline is that it is also a neurotransmitter **(MB Kh Berecek, JM Brody, 1982)**. This hormone is released into the blood under stress conditions and causes increased heartbeats, blood pressure, airway dilation and body preparation for massive energy production, so under these circumstances, the immune system will be deactivated because it is a great energy consumer.

Once this hormone released into the body will cause the extremities of the limbs to become cold almost instantly precisely because the energies are gathered to react in a high intensity moment.

At the level of central nervous system, adrenaline becomes an activating neurotransmitter triggered by neurobehavioral GABA inhibitors to take one of the three instinctual decisions, namely to flee, to freeze or to fight in an imminent dangerous situation. That brings us to the following questions: would GABA neurotransmitters play a role in those mnesic awakenings of the Alzheimer's patient? Then how is it possible that the patient remains 100% lucid during these awakenings? Maybe because that specific intensity of fear is not reached under these circumstances. This type of fear is not the same kind perceived by traditional senses, it is something above that, something like from within the soul. This kind of phenomenon is very developed in animals, would that be the sixth sense? Well, it is a possibility.

In the case of other patients suffering from Alzheimer's disease in the terminal phase, adrenaline causes a state of excitation of neuronal transmissions and, thus, memory can be re-accessed, but certain mechanisms of language are already severely impaired and cannot adequately communicate but the look in their eyes, as well as tears induce us the fact that they understand what is happening in those moments. Let's not forget that ability of speech and breathing are affected last in this disease. As we have previously shown, one can live without amygdalae even hippocampus but not without the hypothalamus or brain stem because among many other things it regulates the autonomic nervous system. That's why in terminal phase an Alzheimer's patient has respiratory problems and dies because the brain stem is severely affected.

That being said, we infer that we are dealing with a severe distortion of the amygdala, basal ganglia, hypothalamus, brain stem mechanisms of investment with emotional values of stimuli, responses or both that, sometimes, they keep returning to optimal functionality. Here can be added also the possibility that the hippocampus cannot correctly pass on the input information or even the output response correctly or not at all. Could it be a greater need for energy in the region of the entorhinal cortex and this will give the impulse necessary for the functioning of the neurons remaining in activity in the hippocampus and amygdala and in the same time in gyrus dentatus to boost the neurogenesis? We tend to believe this possibility as well...

According to the effects of adrenaline such as mnesic awakening of patients in the terminal phase, we must influence our guidelines for possible treatment to stop the degeneration of Alzheimer's disease and why not the healing of patients at a relatively young age (around 50) that would allow a possibility to regenerate affected parts of the brain. This does not mean that in order to cure a patient, will need to be pumped with adrenaline, no, we only need to study the mechanisms triggered by this hormone to be able to fully understand the mnesic awakenings.

We strongly believe that this disease can be cured sooner or later.

As mentioned during our work, at the moment, the treatment for Alzheimer's sufferers has a symptomatic character because its ontogenesis is not well known yet. So the focus is so far on treating the symptoms and slowing as far as possible the degeneration of the patient's pathological conditions but...we have the information that on 6th October 2014, American researchers at the University of California, Los Angeles (UCLA) have managed to restore the memory of patients after a period of three to six months through an ultra-healthy customised treatment (exactly what we were saying in our new paradigm approach towards patient-centred treatment) without any medication.

The author of this study, Doctor in Neuroscience, Dale Bredesen, in partnership with the Buck Institute for Research and Aging, has shown that nine out of ten patients affected by memory loss due to Alzheimer's have recovered after applying an ultra-healthy ***treatment centred on the patient***.

That includes the following:

- Elimination of carbohydrates, gluten and processed foods from diet.
- Higher consumption of vegetables, fruit and fish fished in nature and not from farms.
- Yoga and meditation.
- Increase in sleep duration of, at least, seven hours per night.
- At least, 30 minutes of physical exercise seven days a week.
- Vitamin supplement according to blood analysis but without prescription of medicines.

Although there were significant improvements in one patient, it could not be fully recovered because the disease was too advanced in his case.

However, Dr Bredesen said that this treatment is just a finger in the water because it needs more patients and more documentation to say that it is the best treatment, but it is a beginning which is very important.

We are adepts of this treatment before any other intervention measure on patients in the early or moderate phase of Alzheimer's disease which shows, indeed, that Alzheimer's is an illness of the whole body. That leads us once again to the Thracian paradigm of medicine generated a couple of thousands of years ago by Zalmoxis teachings saying…"You cannot treat the head without treating the body…" This Zalmoxian kind of thinking, fortunately rediscovered, has generated a new type of medicine today called *integrative medicine* which is taking account on the whole person including his environmental lifestyle.

In conclusion, we can say that Alzheimer's disease is not a central nervous system disease but a whole-body disease as we said above in which triggering factors are encountered in the bio-psycho-socio-cultural system from our living environment. From this idea, a new concept was generated called **_epigenetic control_** in which perception of the environment, influence and controls our genetics.

"The mind cannot be occupied by positive and negative emotions at the same time. It has to predominate either some or the others. It is our responsibility to make sure that positive emotions are the ones that dominate the mind."
– Napoleon Hill

Chapter IV. Conclusions

We begin this chapter in the company's words full of wisdom of American author of personal development thinking, Napoleon Hill (1883–1970) regarding the management of emotions.

As it is well known, emotions can be negative or positive, and they alternate according to the orientation of human thinking in relation to external factors from the environment.

Human thinking occurs at all levels of awareness, predominantly at the conscious level. Depending on the experiences of more or less important events, an emotional value loading of different intensities is attributed to these thoughts.

This emotional value load is attributed to representations. Representations differ from a person to another depending on individual or collective experiences.

The ratio between negative and positive experiences is the 21/1 in favour of the first, unfortunately, according to studies at Harvard University done over a period of 75 years. A very important thing to mention here is how much of emotional load and at what intensity are those negative experiences interpreted by the brain of an individual.

If unpleasant experiences are heavily loaded emotionally for a too long period of time, they will in the long run affect the neuroendocrine system, especially the adrenal glands, which in stressful conditions increase their hormone production of adrenaline and cortisol.

The body responds to stress through the path called the stress axis, described for the first time by Hans Selye:

- Hypothalamus
- Hypophysis
- Thyroid
- Adrenals

The body has the ability to adapt, but there is a good chance that this adaptability will no longer normalise in terms of reversibility in cases of prolonged stress, so it becomes chronical

This will generate the so-called *General Adaptation Syndrome*. This theory belongs to one of the greatest endocrinologists of the world, namely Janos Hugo Bruno Hans Selye (1907–1982). This researcher of Austro – Hungarian origin was the first to demonstrate the existence of biological stress.

Selye has deduced through his research that stress is the major cause of illnesses because chronic stress causes long-term chemical changes in the body.

It can be said that Alzheimer's disease has an ontogenesis in the stress caused by the environment of the individual, so, eventually, it becomes a disease of the whole body.

In conclusion, we remain in the opinion that the best intervention regarding the treatment of patients with Alzheimer's dementia is the personalised treatment of the sufferer according to the results of the individual analyses.

We are not in favour of treatment 'in mass', practiced in most of the clinics across the globe because it is cheaper which, in our opinion, is kind of stereotypical as well. Therefore, we firmly support the project of American Doctor of Neuroscience Dale Bredesen of Los Angeles University in California regarding the strictly and ultra-healthy treatment described previously.

However, we should mention that this type of treatment should be applied in the incipient phase of Alzheimer's disease in a specialised clinic for a period of several months, after which, it will be continued rigorously at home throughout the rest of their life.

We consider it of the outmost importance that the patient, when the applied treatment reaches optimal rates of physical and mental functioning in accordance with his age, before leaving the clinic will have to have a personalised profile of the blood, urine and cerebrospinal fluid analysis in order to serve as an ***optimal reference point.***

The optimal point of reference that differs from one person to another is the standard for achieving the patient's optimal physical and psychological performance.

This reference point needs to be checked in the beginning every six months and subjected to ***fine-tuning*** if necessary.

If a certain value of an element of the analysis result deviates from the reference point; for example, a deficiency or deviation of vitamins, proteins, certain hormonal values, etc., there will be taking place the so-called fine-tuning by which it is understood a restoration of deficient or deviant conditions.

The benefits of this way of patient intervention and supervision not only make the individual recover to society gaining back its normal functionality, which is the overriding reason, but patient care costs are significantly reduced on the long run both financially and especially emotionally because more people are involved around a case like that.

Because by this disease, large number of individuals are being affected, the governments should do more about this problem like unlocking a larger amount of money for research in order to cure it. Another thing the governments should do is to watch over the quality of alimentation of their population because there are so many things out there bad for people because of greed of certain companies from food and beverage industries. Pollution is another thing the governments should really do something about it. People should have more free time to proper educate their kids and/or recharge their batteries in order to perform better in their jobs. Because people spend most of their active time at work place, they should be provided with a healthy work climate free of mobbing or emotional abuse at work place because this is a very big problem too at the moment.

It is a moral and ethical duty of the governments to take good care of the health of their people that is why they are voted and elected by the masses.

In our view, the more members of a society have a lower level of stress, the healthier the society will be, and with this idea, we finish this work that we hope will be well received by our readers.

Bibliography

Bruce D Perry – *The boy who was raised as a dog pg. 125 – 134 Editura Basic Books USA New York, 2006.*
Barry Reisberg – *Guide to Alzheimer's disease, pg. 23–28, Free press. USA NewYork, 1984.*
Carl W Cotman – *Behavioural neuroscience, pg. 173–189, Kindle edition. USA New York, 2014.*
Dick Swaab – *Wij zijn ons brein pg 50, editura Atlas Contact Uitgeverij NL Amsterdam, 2010.*
Elena C Rusu – *Psihologie cognitivă, editura România de Mâine. Bucureşti, 2008*
Golu, Mihai – *Fundamentele Psihologiei vol.1, pg. 166–167, editura România de Mâine. Bucureşti, 2007.*
Graţiela Sion – *Psihologia Vârstelor, editura România de Mâine, Bucureşti, 2007*
Lungu, Nicolae – *Psihologie experimentală, editura România de Mâine, Bucureşti, 2008*
Manfred Spitzer – *Digitale Dementie, Droemer Verlag, NL Steenwijk, 2013*
Rene Kahn – *Onze hersenen pg. 39–40; 46 editura Uitgeverij Balans, NL Amsterdam, 2006*
Stanciu, Corneliu – *Introducere în psihofiziologie pg. 45 editura România de Mâine,Bucureşti, 2009.*
Tudose, Florin – *Psihopatologie şi orientări terapeutice în psihiatrie pg 234 editura România de Mâine, 2009.*

Other Publications

Is het dementie? Pg. 23–33 uitgeverij Alzheimer Nederland 2013

Daily Mail Telegraph 06-11-2012

Magazin istoric, anul III, Nr 4 (25), aprilie 1969

De Volkskrant 29-09-2016

Web Resources

http://www.hln.be/hln/nl/17541/Het-leukste-van-het-web/article/detail/2025361/2014/09/02/Ontroerend-mama-met-Alzheimer-herkent-even-haar-dochter.dhtml

http://www.khou.com/story/news/health/2014/10/06/study-memory-loss-from-alzheimers-reversed/16839173/

https://www.alzheimer.nl/over-alzheimer/herkennen-en-behandelen

http://www.btsg.nl/infobulletin/dementie/dementie-neuropsychologisch.html

http://www.apotheek.nl/Medische_informatie/Medicijnen/Producten/Rivastigmine.aspx?mId=10704&rId=2572#L1

http://en.wikipedia.org/wiki/NMDA_receptor

http://www.brainmatters.nl/terms/substantia-nigra/

http://en.wikipedia.org/wiki/Tau_protein

http://dreamhawk.com/dream-encyclopedia/brain-levels-and-dreams/

https://www.ncbi.nlm.nih.gov/pmc/articles/PMC3277080/

http://en.wikibooks.org/wiki/Human_Physiology/Senses

http://hipporeads.com/plato-studied-in-africa-the-case-for-culturally-inclusive-philosophy/

https://www.epilepsy.com/connect/forums/surgery-and-devices/right-temporal-lobe-surgery-removal-right-hippocampus

https://www.ncbi.nlm.nih.gov/pmc/articles/PMC3587151/

https://www.wired.com/2014/05/heres-what-happens-when-a-neurosurgeon-slurps-out-your-hippocampus/

https://www.ncbi.nlm.nih.gov/pmc/articles/PMC4210314/
http://neurosciencenews.com/sm-fearless-woman-missing-amygdala/

https://en.wikipedia.org/wiki/Mitochondrion

http://www.sfatulmedicului.ro/Stresul-si-sindromul-de-oboseala-cronica/stresul-oxidativ_11554

http://www.pnas.org/content/early/2018/03/29/1721694115

https://www.physiology.org/doi/abs/10.1152/ajpregu.1990.259.5.R943

https://www.bbc.com/news/health-19093442

https://en.wikipedia.org/wiki/Genesis_flood_narrative

CPSIA information can be obtained
at www.ICGtesting.com
Printed in the USA
LVHW051318250420
654423LV00011B/211

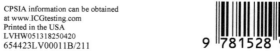

9 781528 979849